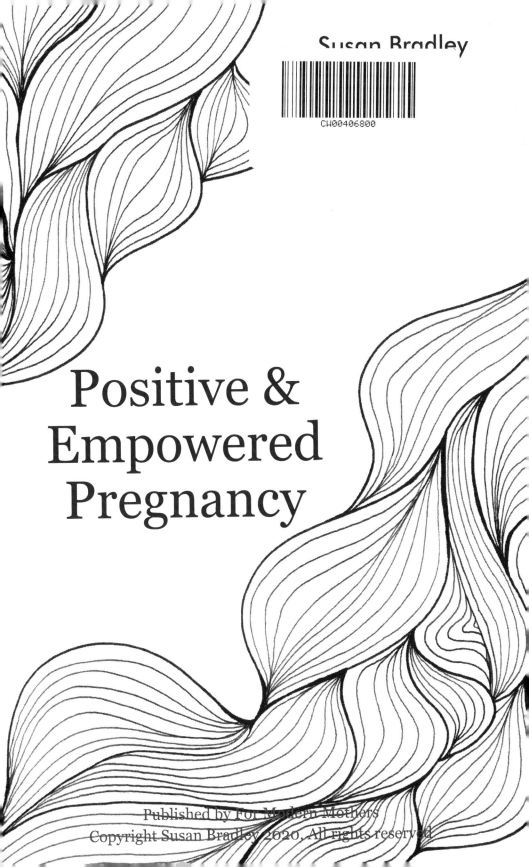

Susan Bradley

CW00406800

Positive &
Empowered
Pregnancy

Published by For Modern Mothers

About the author

Susan Bradley is a celebrated British designer who for over 15 years has been as a creative director on numerous products, interior projects, and large scale installations. Working with companies including Donna Karan New York, Selfridges, Christian Louboutin, Yorkshire Sculpture Park, Southbank Centre and London Transport Museum.

Susan's designs have won international acclaim being sold and exhibited around the world and winning a number of awards. Her distinctive graphic work has encompassed furniture design, interior and exterior accessories, installations, products, pattern design and lighting - and now a book.

Her love of pattern, colour and typography informs this book. Particularly from the pared back design traditions of Scandinavia and Japan. Marrying simplicity with strong bold designs.

For the past seven years she has also been working with women empowering their journey into and through motherhood. Susan draws from her vast professional experience as a pregnancy and postnatal yoga teacher, an antenatal educator and hypnobirthing teacher, doula and women's self-care advocate to bring you this unique book. It's aim is to help you have a more positive, mindful, creative and empowered pregnancy. To celebrate all that you are in a positive way, and boost your self belief and confidence through your pregnancy and into labour.

About this book

This book is a bringing together of Susans expertise and her passions. Creating a simple yet effective way to give you time to mindfully be present and connect with your pregnancy and your baby in a calm, positive and empowering way. We know that colouring in can be a great way to have some relaxing me-time, and this book gives you that opportunity specifically in your pregnancy.

The designs are created by hand, lo-fi, using ink on paper. There are purposeful imperfections that have been left in the designs, they have not been 'airbrushed' by a computer. This is intentional and is part of their charm. Because airbrushing life is not real life. Honouring and savouring what is real, true and honest makes far more sense, it is more human and more charming. Because life is perfectly imperfect, and that should be celebrated.

There are also a few affirmations at end of the book with space for you to draw you own doodles and patterns, to create your own unique piece of affirmation art. Simply make some marks, be bold, aim for something unique - not something perfect. Embrace creating something for enjoyment, for fun, and allow yourself time to relax a little too.

About Positive Affirmations

This book is combines pattern with positive words or 'affirmations'. As you colour the words and patterns, and your mind relaxes into the moment let these positive statements sink in. Then you can keep them together in the book, or carefully cut them from their binding and put them up around your home to help bring positivity about pregnancy, labour and birth into your days.

By doing this you create a simple habit of positive thoughts, helping to shift your mindset. The more you tell yourself something, the more you believe it, and the more you live by it. Through the journey of pregnancy, and into labour and birth a little daily positive reprogramming of your sub-conscious mind, with these little daily bursts of positivity, can help you to grow your inner confidence and self-belief. Giving you calmness and confidence in navigating your path to parenthood. Simple yet so powerful.

You could also take a photograph and use it as your phone or computer screen saver. And don't forget to put them up in your birth space and pack some into your hospital bag to use there too.

If one really resonates with you, you can use it as your personal mantra and keep repeating it through your pregnancy and labour too.

You can also listen to an audio track of positive affirmations that I have recorded to go alongside this book. To receive a complimentary Positive Affirmations For Pregnancy MP3 head to my website and download for free here:

www.formodernmothers com/positivepregnancybook

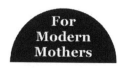

For
Modern
Mothers

Pick up a colour, relax and have fun

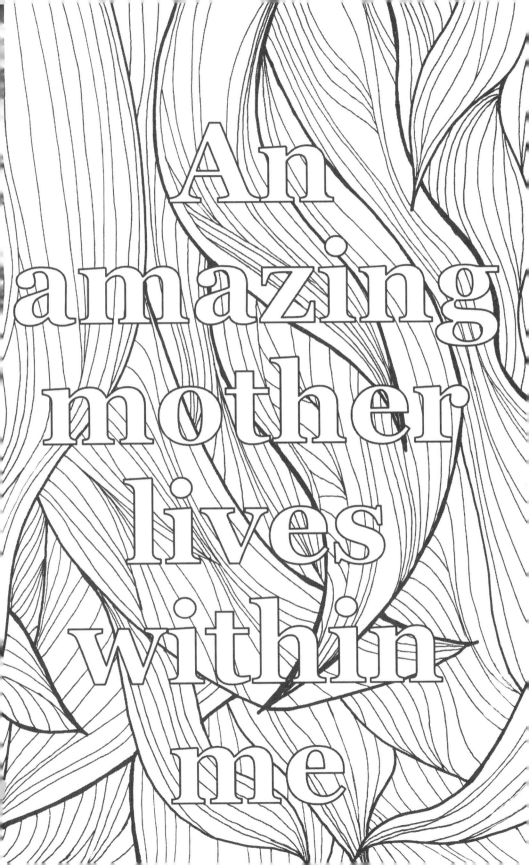

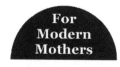

For
Modern
Mothers

An amazing mother lives within me

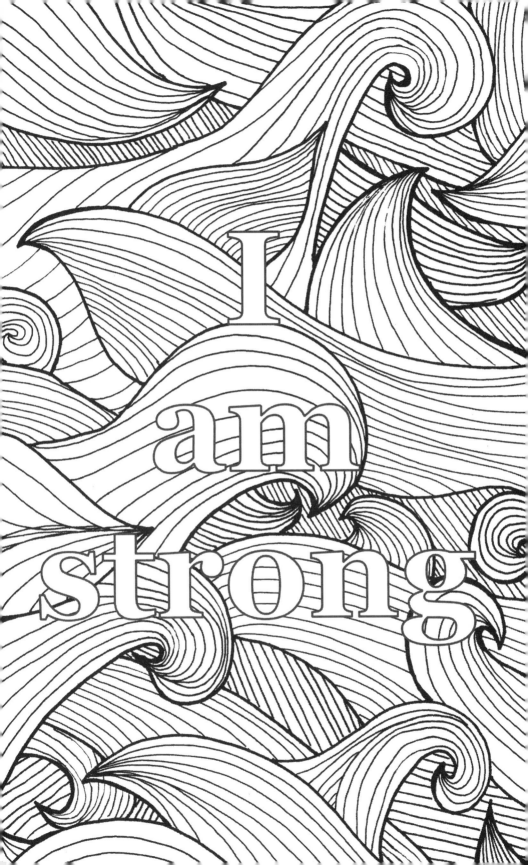

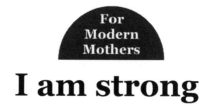

For
Modern
Mothers

I am strong

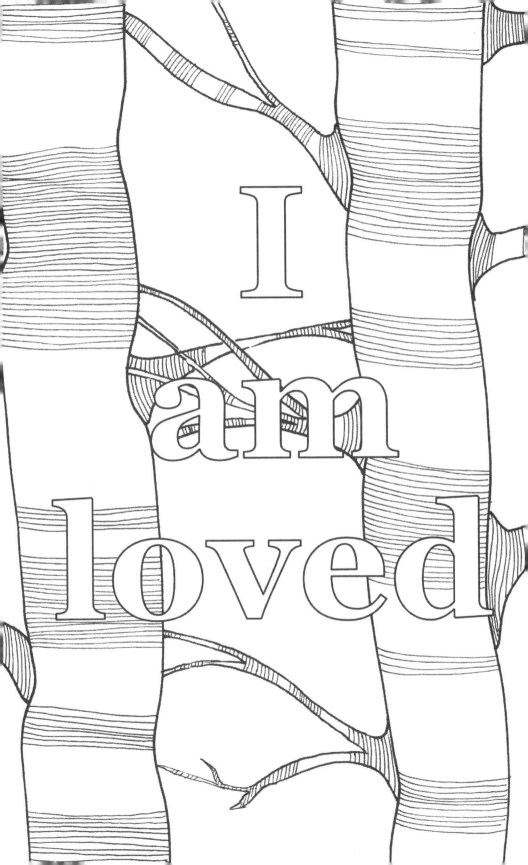

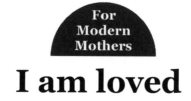

For
Modern
Mothers

I am loved

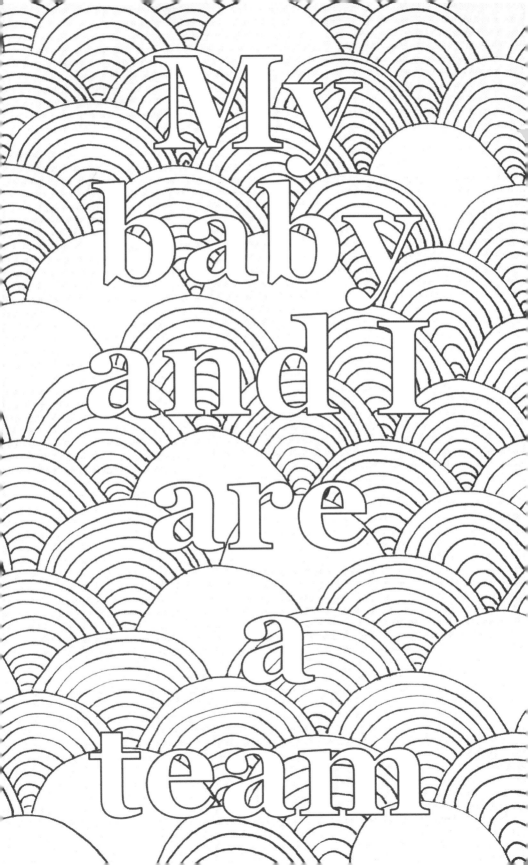

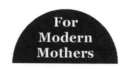

My baby and I are a team

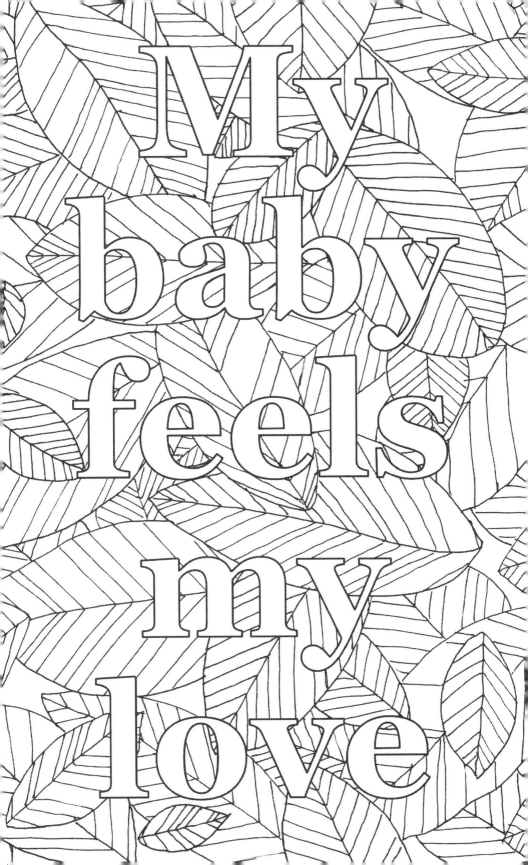

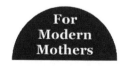

For
Modern
Mothers

My baby feels my love

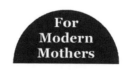

For Modern Mothers

I honour my changing body

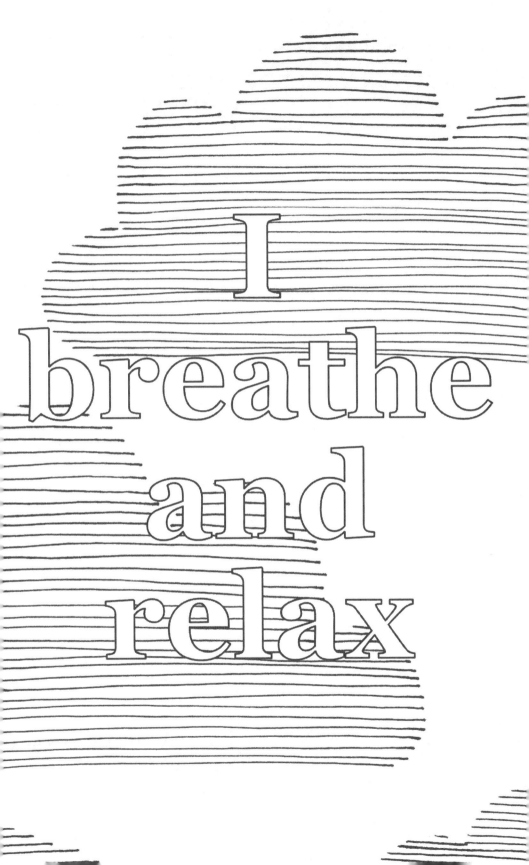

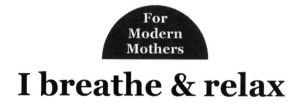

For
Modern
Mothers

I breathe & relax

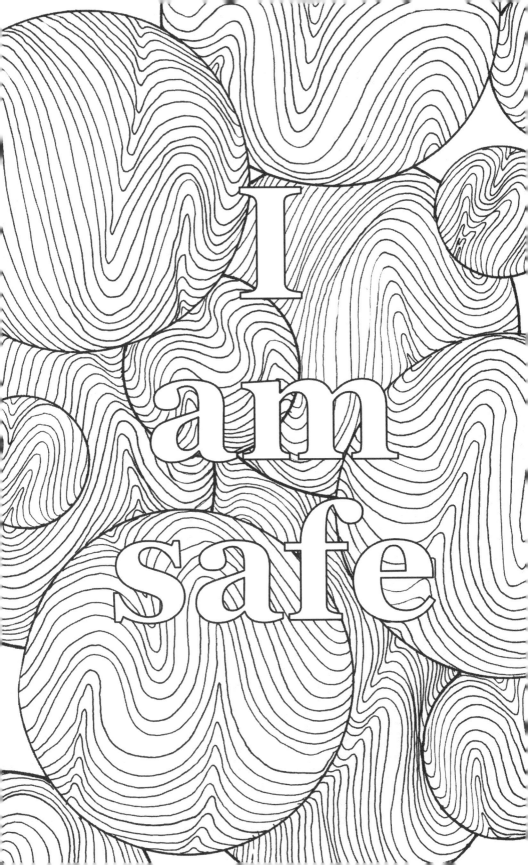

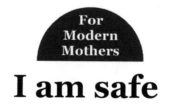

For
Modern
Mothers

I am safe

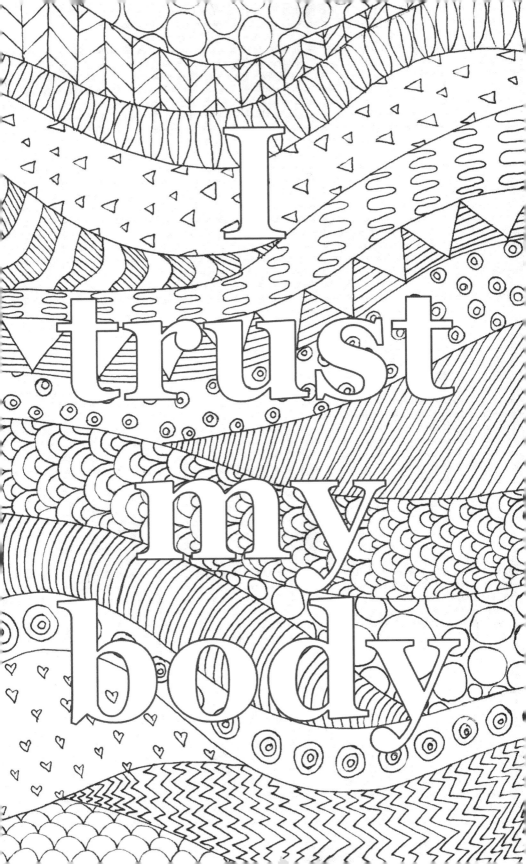

I trust my body

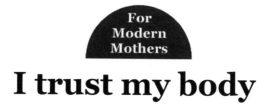

For Modern Mothers

I trust my body

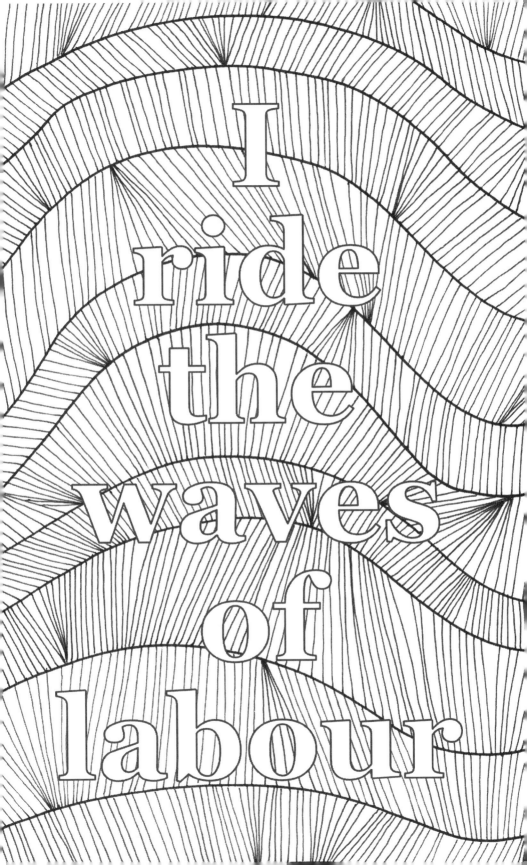

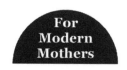

I ride the waves of labour

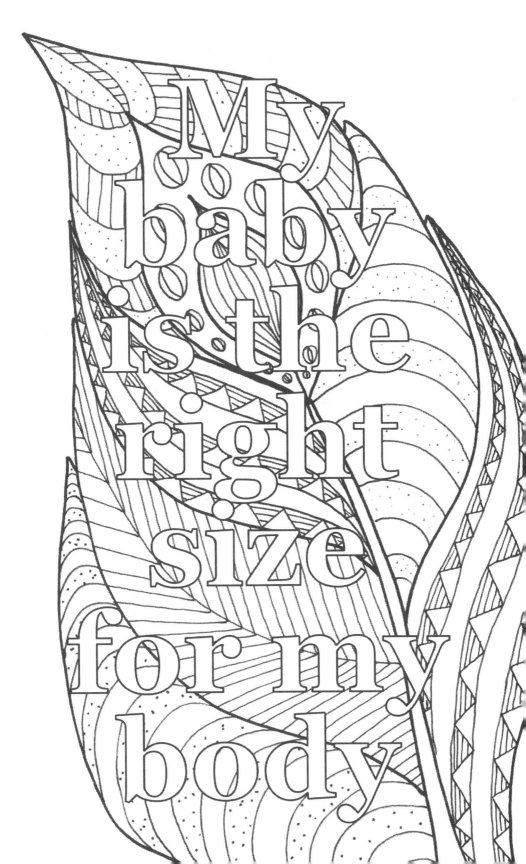

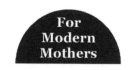

My baby is the right size for my body

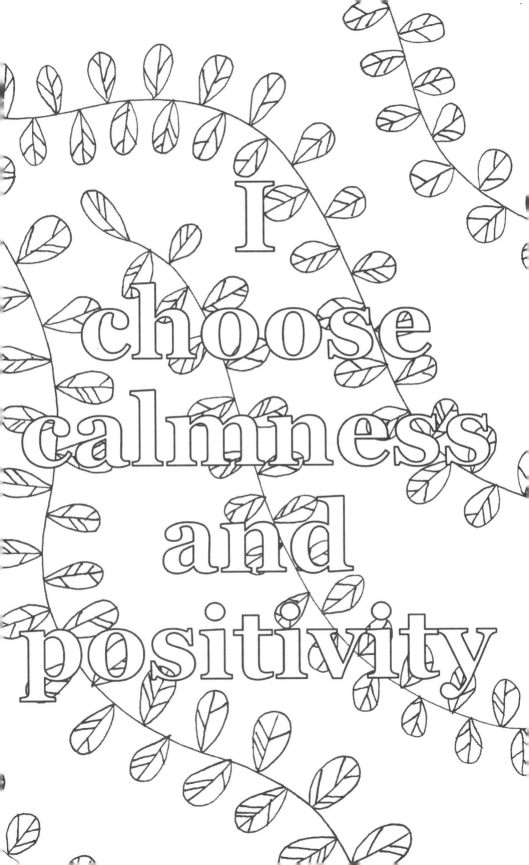

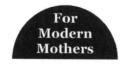

For
Modern
Mothers

I choose calmness and positivity

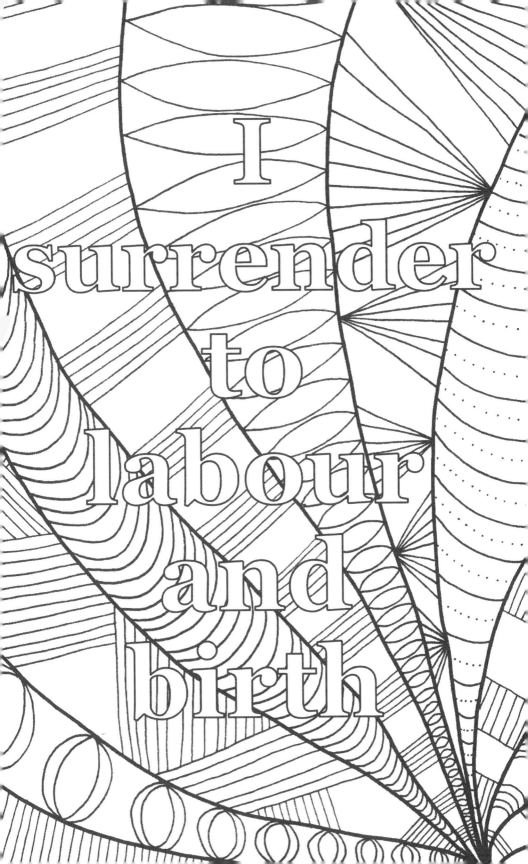

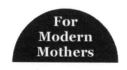

I surrender to labour

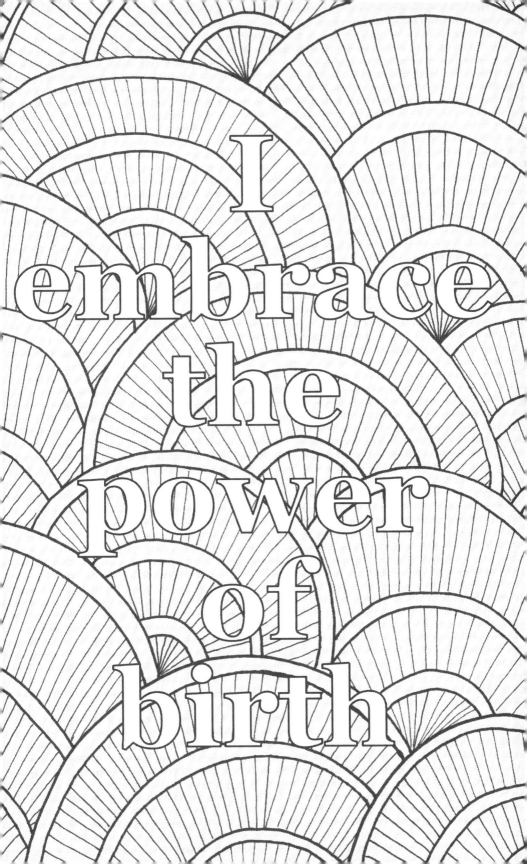

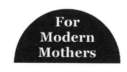

For
Modern
Mothers

I embrace the power of birth

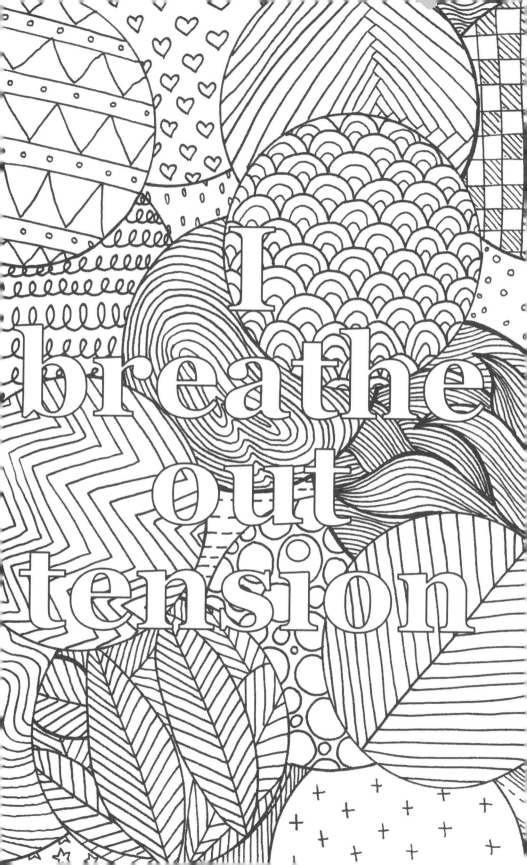

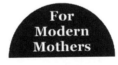

For
Modern
Mothers

I breathe out tension

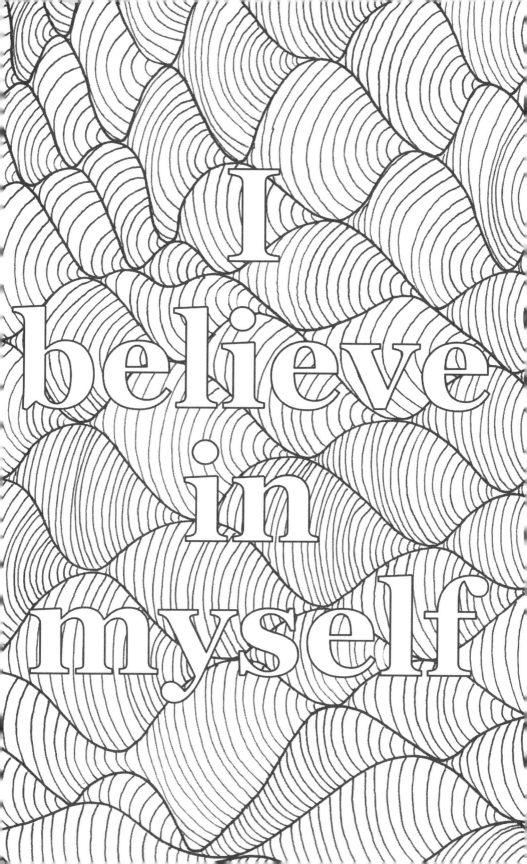

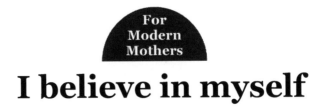

For Modern Mothers

I believe in myself

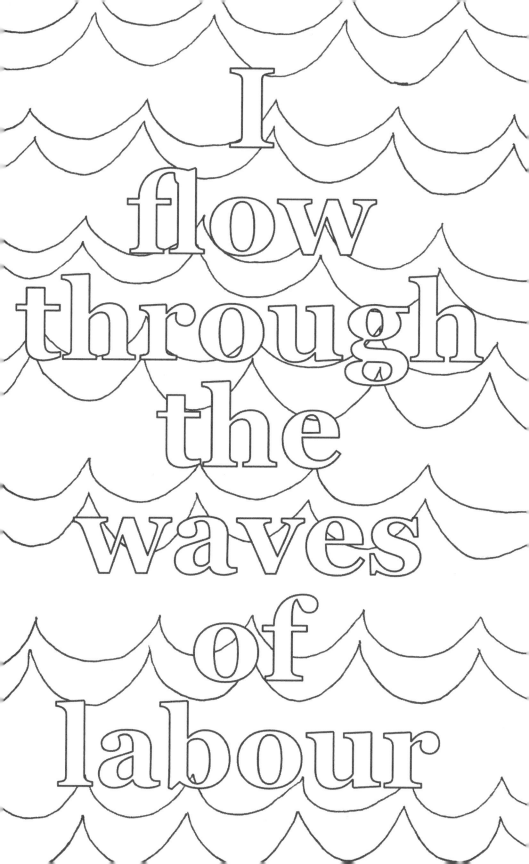

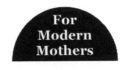

For
Modern
Mothers

I flow through the waves of labour

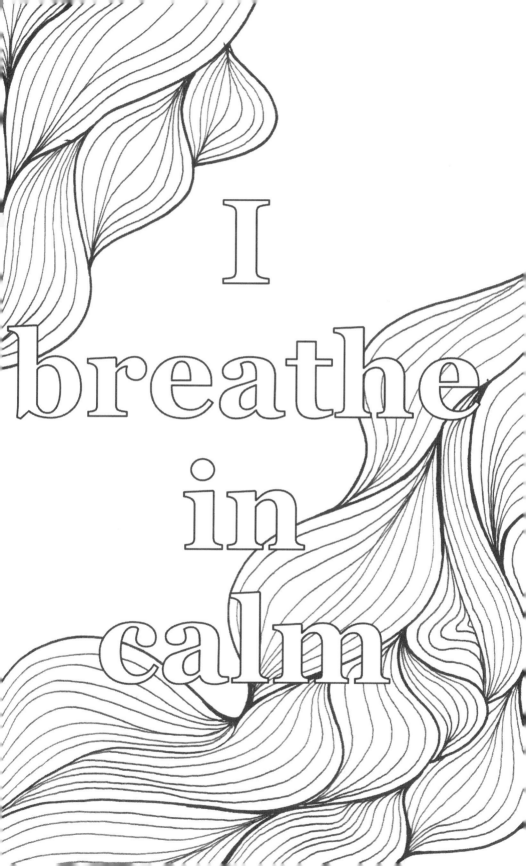

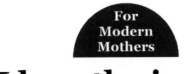

For
Modern
Mothers

I breathe in calm

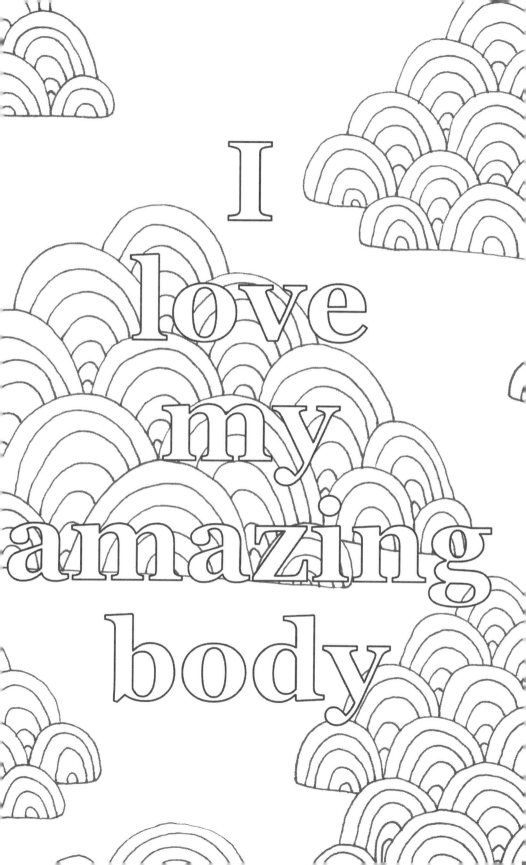

I love my amazing body

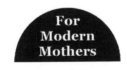

For
Modern
Mothers

I love my amazing body

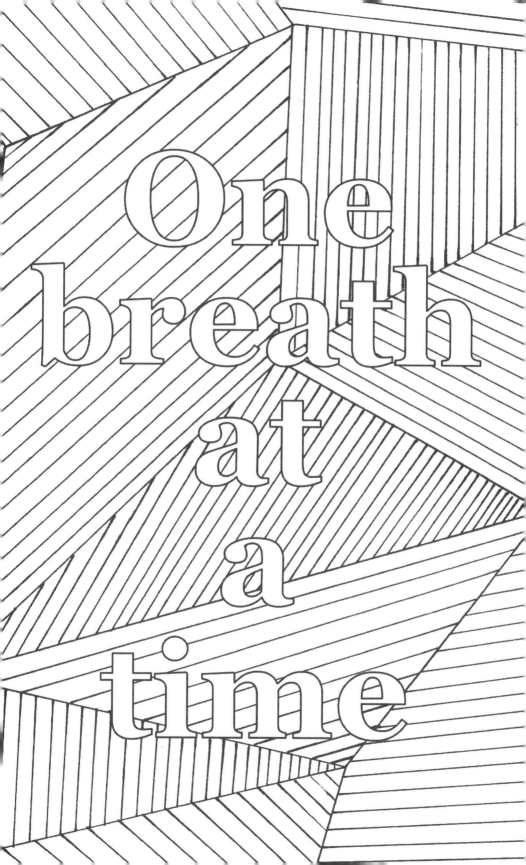

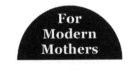

One breath at a time

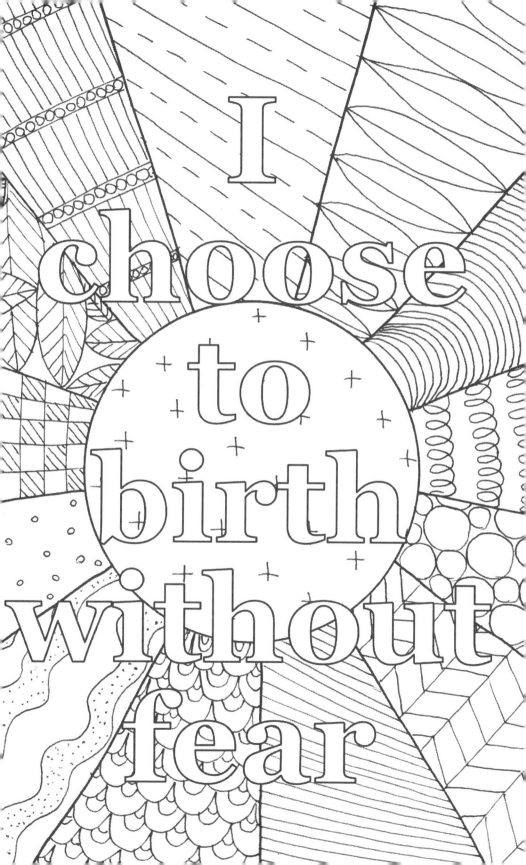

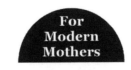

I choose to birth without fear

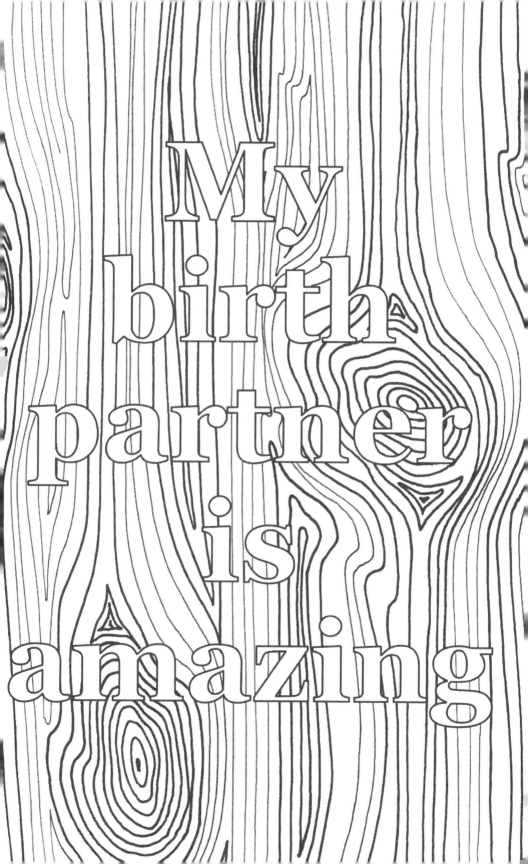

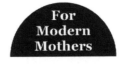

For Modern Mothers

My birth partner is amazing

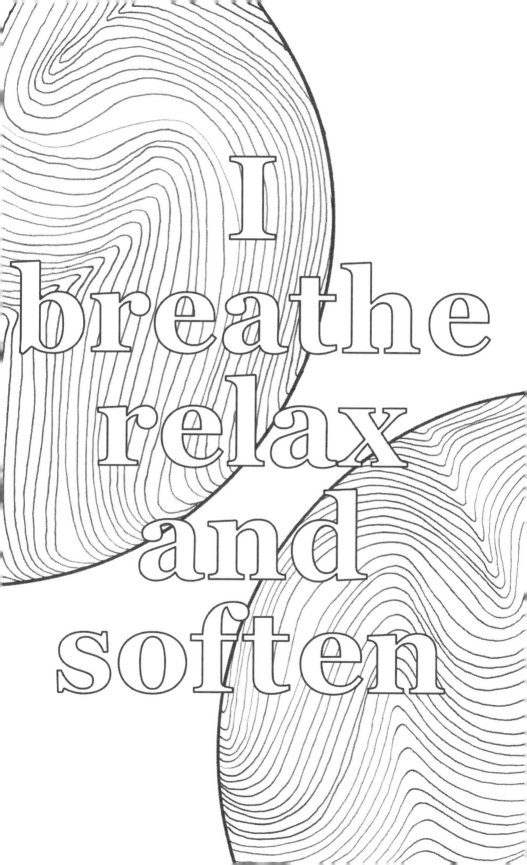

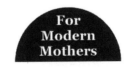

For
Modern
Mothers

I breathe, relax and soften

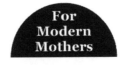

For
Modern
Mothers

I feel safe and loved

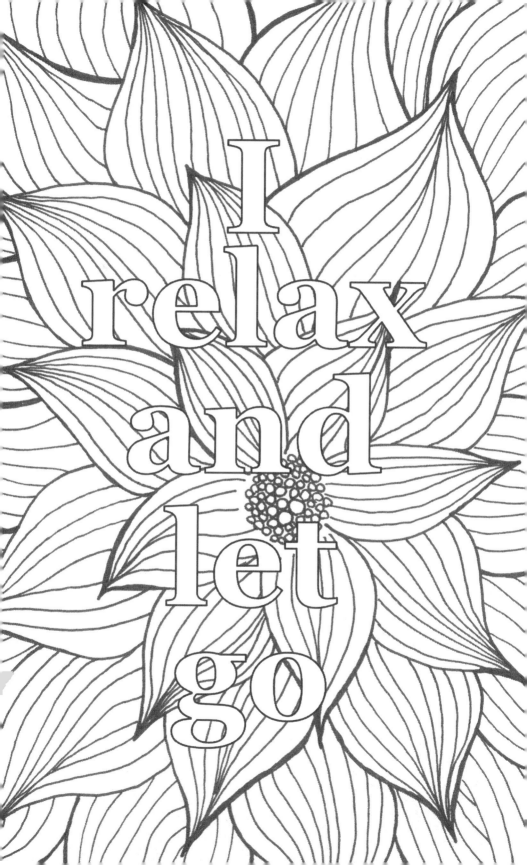

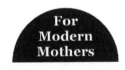

For Modern Mothers

Over to you. Get doodling....

I
have
strength
&
courage

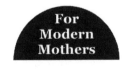

For Modern Mothers

Design your own affirmations

I
breathe
in
love

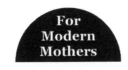

Play, have fun, feel free

I connect to my birth instincts